THE URGENT
INVERSION

THE URGENT INVERSION

From the PEN of a LAYPERSON

CAROL CURTIS

iUniverse, Inc.
New York   Bloomington

The information, ideas, and suggestions in this book are not intended as a substitute for professional medical advice. Before following any suggestions contained in this book, you should consult your personal physician. Neither the author nor the publisher shall be liable or responsible for any loss or damage allegedly arising as a consequence of your use or application of any information or suggestions in this book.

iUniverse books may be ordered through booksellers or by contacting:

iUniverse
1663 Liberty Drive
Bloomington, IN 47403
www.iuniverse.com
1-800-Authors (1-800-288-4677)

Because of the dynamic nature of the Internet, any Web addresses or links contained in this book may have changed since publication and may no longer be valid. The views expressed in this work are solely those of the author and do not necessarily reflect the views of the publisher, and the publisher hereby disclaims any responsibility for them.

ISBN: 978-1-4401-6096-7 (sc)
ISBN: 978-1-4401-6095-0 (ebook)
ISBN: 978-1-4401-6094-3 (dj)

Printed in the United States of America

iUniverse rev. date: 9/16/2009

This book is dedicated to the memory of my dear Aunt Vivian, who inspired me to strive for the best, along with my Uncle Jim, Dr. James L. Curtis.

Contents

Acknowledgments

I would like to thank Wilma Skinner, a colleague, for advising me during my first year of teaching to "do something to keep physically fit." I am thankful to God that I had the wisdom to take her advice. I would like to thank Marion Hood for coming into my life and introducing me to yoga. I will never forget the exhilaration that I felt up to three days after she had taken me to a yoga class at the Sivananda Yoga Vedanta Centre in Toronto, Ontario. I would like to thank Doris Epstein for telling me about a yoga class that was within walking distance of my home. I would like to thank my yoga instructor, Axel Molema, for his words of wisdom and for believing in me when I wasn't sure whether I would be able to do the headstand. I would also like to thank my yoga instructor, Svetlana Vasic, for her warmth, encouragement, and advice. I would like to thank Joel Osteen for his words of encouragement and divine inspiration, from which I found the courage to write this book. I would like to thank Dr. Sanjay Gupta, the neurosurgeon, for bringing a greater awareness to Alzheimer's disease, which prompted me to write this book. I would like to thank Wayne Franson, of Back and Body Solutions, for writing his in-depth article on the benefits of inversion therapy devices. I would like to thank my husband, Matthew, for his encouragement to write this book, and my two children, Yusef and Alika, for their help in pulling everything together. I would like to thank the photographer, Nick Basiuk. I would also like to thank Yusef and my brother, Warren, for their photography. I would not have been able to do it without you.

Preface

Over the past twenty plus years, colleagues, friends, and family members have told me that my physical appearance has changed very little. Sometimes they ask me what my secret is. I tell them that I have been consistently doing yoga, particularly the inversion of the brain and heart, for a few minutes daily. When I had my last annual physical, at the age of fifty-seven, my doctor told me that I had the blood pressure of a twenty-year-old. I feel that everyone deserves to enjoy the same benefits that I have been enjoying. It is my responsibility as an educator to write this book, so that I can share with you my research, knowledge, and experience.

Introduction

Would you like to improve the quality of your life and increase your chances of living twenty minutes longer? Would you like to improve the quality of your life and increase your chances of living twenty days longer? Would you like to improve the quality of your life and increase your chances of living twenty years longer? If you have answered in the affirmative to the preceding questions, it is urgent that you take a close look at the two invisible forces of time and gravity. Time and gravity may well be the two most powerful invisible forces of nature. We are aware of the passage of time when we look at a clock or a watch and observe seconds, minutes, and hours passing, and when we see darkness and daylight. We have appointments to keep. The seasons change. We celebrate birthdays, holidays, and religious holy days. With the passage of time, we can see changes in our physical appearance and in the physical appearance of others. We capture moments of time in pictures and videos.

However, it is not nearly as easy to see the force of gravity. If we drop an object or spill a liquid, it falls to the ground. That is because gravity pulls all things, solid or liquid, toward the earth's center. Gravity can be defined as the natural force of attraction between objects at or near the earth's surface, drawing them toward its center. Were it not for the pull of gravity, all liquids and animate and inanimate objects would be weightless, floating. The element of time cannot be stopped, slowed, or reversed. It is an infinite and perpetual force of nature. Gravity, like time, cannot be stopped, but the effects of gravity can be slowed and temporarily reversed.

The combination of the passage of time and the force of gravity is a cause for concern, when we observe their combined effects on the human body. The continuous pull of gravity over time causes the skin, muscles, tissues, and organs of the human body to sag and droop. The facial features drop. Those who can afford it may choose to have a surgical or nonsurgical facelift. We cannot see the effect of gravity and time on our internal organs, but we do know that as we age all functions of the body tend to slow down, including the circulation of the blood.[1]

It is urgent that we take a proactive approach to the cumulative effect of the combined invisible forces of

---

1   Krishna Raman, "Bio-Mechanics of Yoga," <www.medicineau.net.au/columns/yoga/biomech.htm>

gravity and time. We cannot stop these two forces, but we can slow down and reverse their combined effects on the human body.

Here's how: we can position the head lower than the heart. Why is this important? The heart pumps blood throughout the body. When the head is positioned lower than the heart, it is much easier for the heart to pump blood to the brain, because it does not have to work against the pull of gravity. The brain then receives more nourishment and oxygen, as a greater supply of blood is pumped from the heart to the brain. We can enrich our blood by eating foods that contain omega-3 fatty acids, such as cold-water fish, dark green vegetables, and omega-3 oil. When the body is partially or completely inverted, the force of gravity works opposite to the way it normally works on our bodies, and it therefore benefits us, slowing down the aging process.

We usually start life at birth head down. During the last trimester of pregnancy, when the head of the unborn baby is down, there is significant growth and development of the brain.

Alzheimer's Disease

Alzheimer's is a progressive and degenerative disease. The cells of the brain shrink and deteriorate or disappear, causing loss of brain and bodily functions.

The circulation of the blood throughout the body tends to slow down as we become older. The heart has to pump blood to the brain, working up against gravity, and this becomes progressively difficult unless the circulation of the blood to the brain is revitalized.

Studies show that exercise stimulates the flow of blood to the brain, lowering the risk of Alzheimer's.[2] It stands to reason, therefore, that the mild, partial, or full inversion of the brain and heart, which increases the flow of blood to the brain, may help to prevent or alleviate Alzheimer's.

It would be easier for the brain to receive extra oxygen and nourishment carried to it by fresh blood pumped from the heart, when the head is below the

2   Lenore Powell with Katie Courtice. *Alzheimer's Disease: A guide for Families and Caregivers*, 310.

heart. According to research, people who have a family history of Alzheimer's will not necessarily get the disease.[3] The inversion of the brain and heart may also help to prevent or alleviate other disorders of the brain, such as Parkinson's disease,[4] chronic depression, mental illness, and addictions. It may also help to prevent stroke, because certain inverted postures, like the shoulder stand and headstand, lower the blood pressure, bringing it to normal.

---

3   Marwan Noel Sabbagh, *The Alzheimer's Answer*, 74–75 and 189–190.
4   Krishna Raman, "Bio-Mechanics of Yoga," <www. medicineau.net.au/columns/yoga/biomech.htm>

Brain/Heart Inversions

The following are some examples of mild (or partial) inversions and full inversions of the brain and the heart. You should get the consent of your doctor before doing any inversion of the brain and heart. Do what your body allows you to comfortably do. Breathe deeply to maximize the benefits of the inversion. Your stomach should distend when you breathe in and flatten when you breathe out. Inversions can be safely introduced if they are introduced gradually. The mild, (or partial), inversion of the heart and brain can be achieved by anyone. Even those with physical challenges can achieve these, under a doctor's supervision, if necessary. Mild, (or partial), inversions can be introduced before gradually moving to steeper inversions, if desired. The outlined benefits of the following postures are derived from the inversion of the brain and the heart or of the entire body.

Forward Bends

Sitting Forward Bend

Start in a sitting position on a chair.

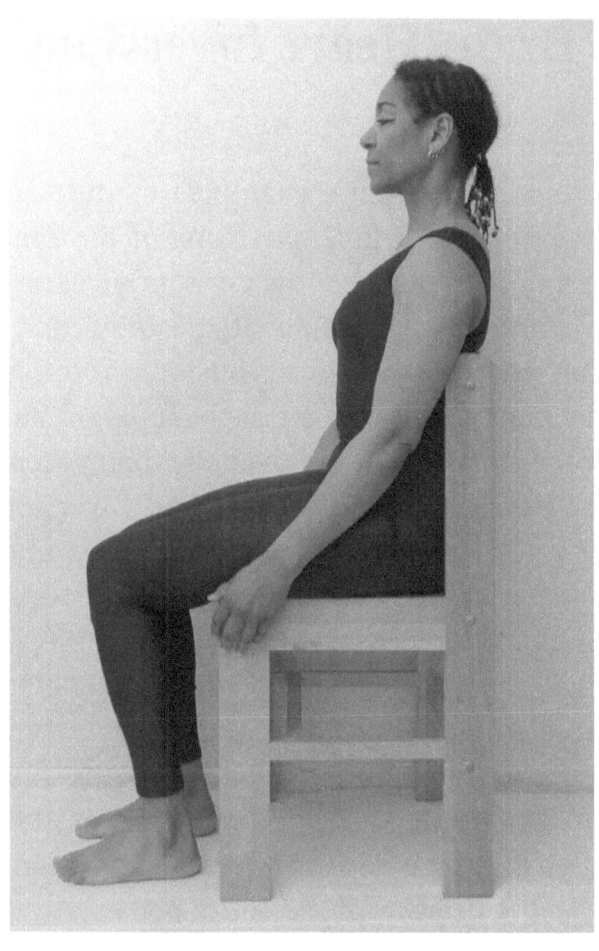

Bend forward slowly, allowing the head to go between the knees and down as far as possible.

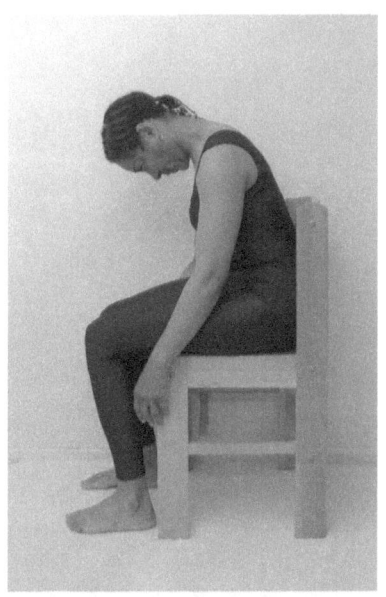

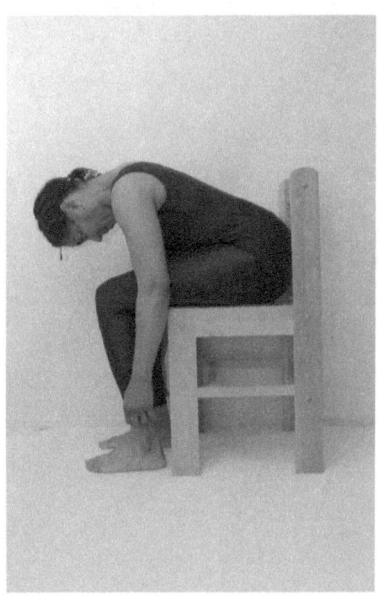

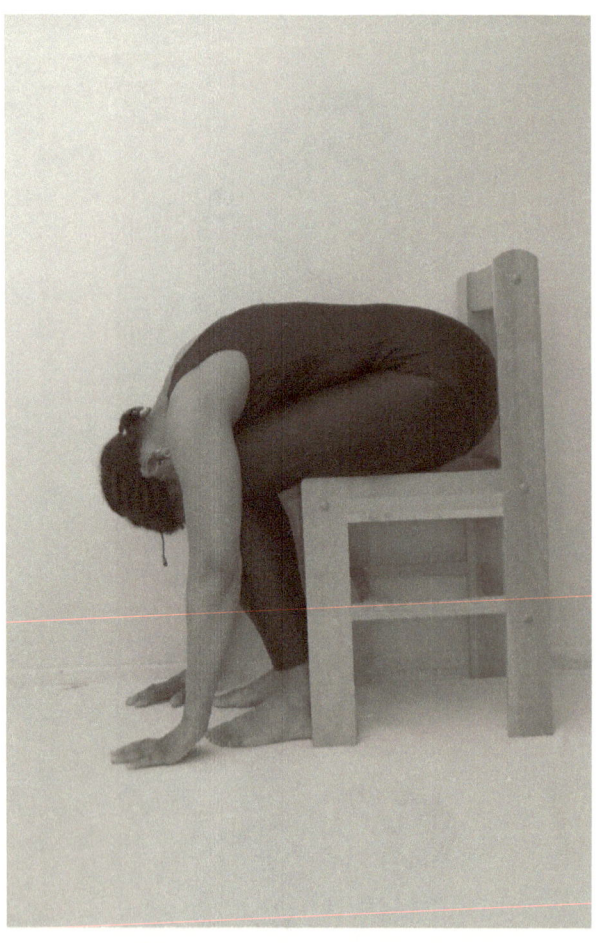

The fingers or palms of the hands should touch the floor. Stay in this position for thirty seconds to one minute.

Slowly come back up to a sitting position.

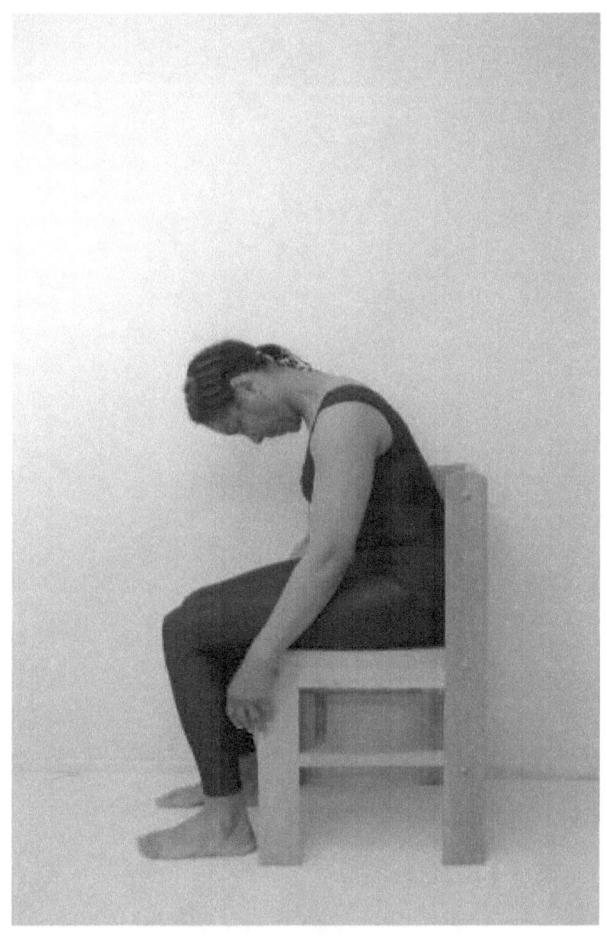

Repeat this exercise two more times.

Standing Forward Bend

Start in a standing position.

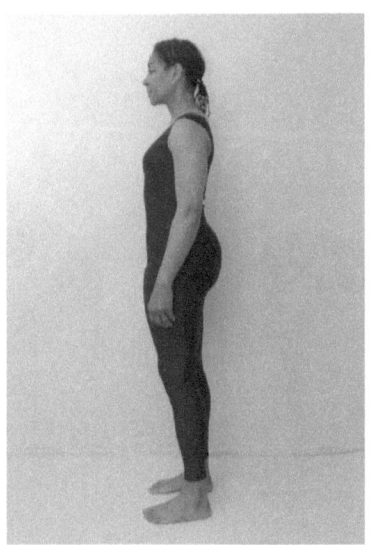

Bend forward at the waist.

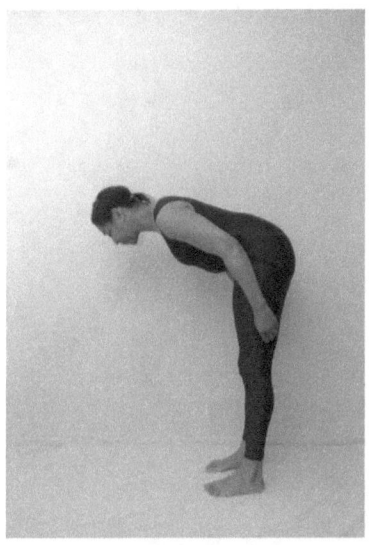

Reach downward toward your toes, as far as possible, with straight arms. Your knees can be straight or slightly bent.

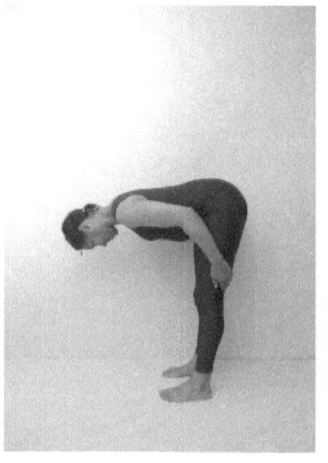 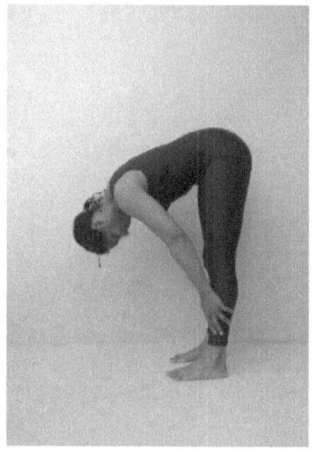

The fingers, or the palms of the hands, if possible, are touching the floor. Look back beyond your legs. Stay in this position for thirty seconds to one minute.

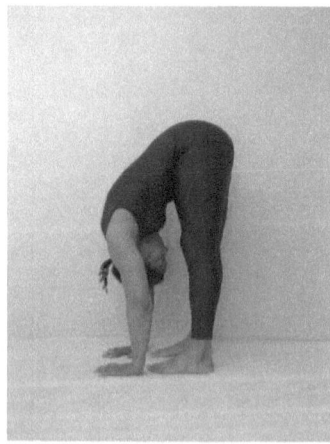

Slowly, one vertebra at a time, come back up to a standing position.

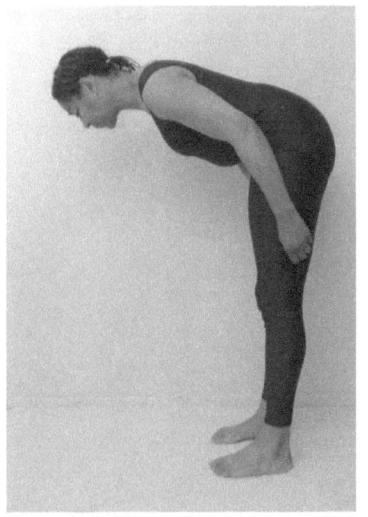 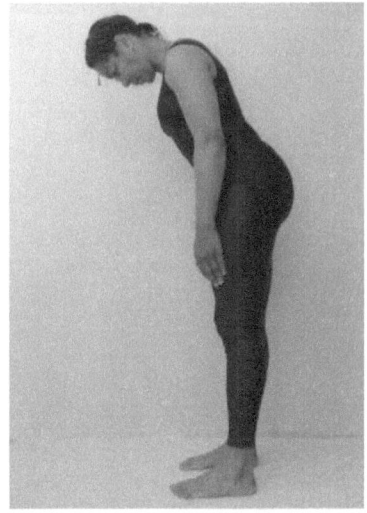

Repeat this exercise two more times.

Benefits of Forward Bends

Forward bends stimulate the flow of blood to the brain, calming the mind.[5]

---

5   Donna Farhi, *Yoga Mind, Body & Spirit: A Return to Wholeness,* 113

Downward Dog
(Adho Mukha Svanasana)

Come to your hands and knees on your mat, with your wrists shoulder distance apart and your upper body parallel to your mat.

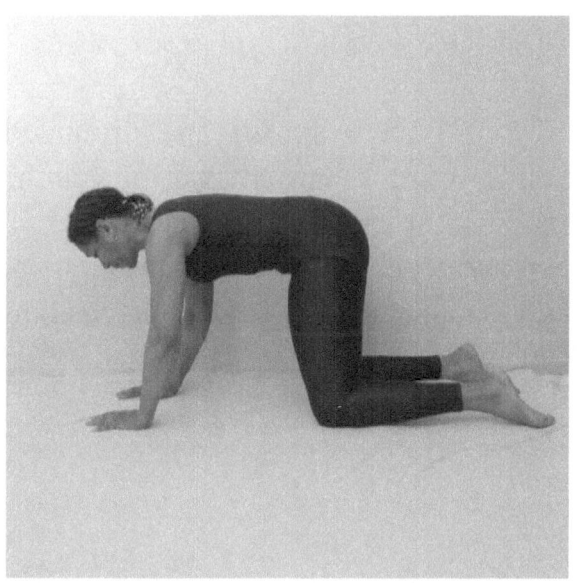

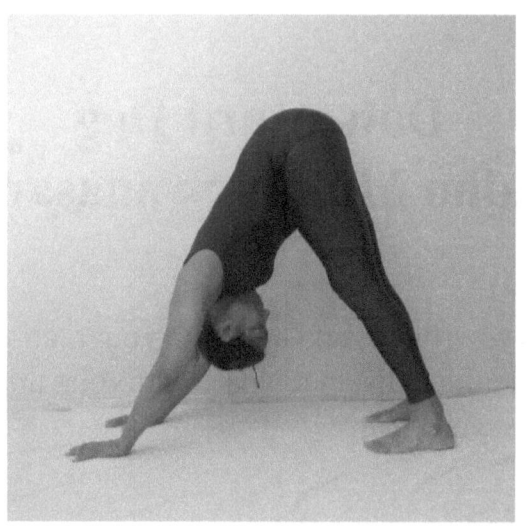

    With your fingers spread and grounded, push back, curling your toes upward, raising your hips, and straightening your legs. Let your head hang.

    Draw your heels as close to your mat as possible. Your body should be in a triangular position. Look back beyond your legs.

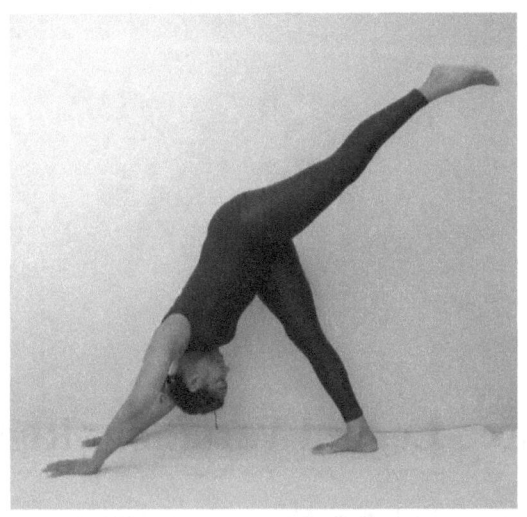

Three-Legged Variation (Left)

Start in Downward Dog position. Raise your left leg backward, as straight and as high as possible. Look back beyond your left leg. Hold for thirty seconds to one minute. Then return the leg to its original position.

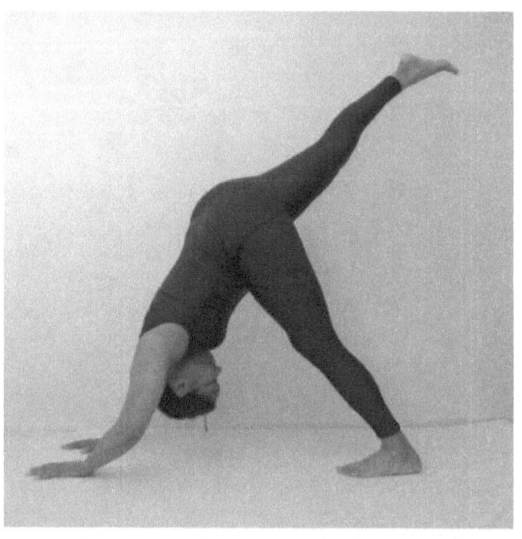

Three-Legged Variation (Right)

Raise your right leg backward as straight and as high as possible. Look back beyond your right leg. Hold for thirty seconds to one minute. Then return the leg to its original position.

Benefits of Downward Dog

The Downward Dog posture, like the shoulder stand and headstand (to follow), eliminates fatigue and rejuvenates the brain cells.[6]

---

6   Krishna Raman, "Bio-Mechanics of Yoga," <www.medicineau.net.au/columns/yoga/biomech.htm> .

Shoulder Stand (Sarvangasana)

On your mat, assume the starting position,
lying on your back.

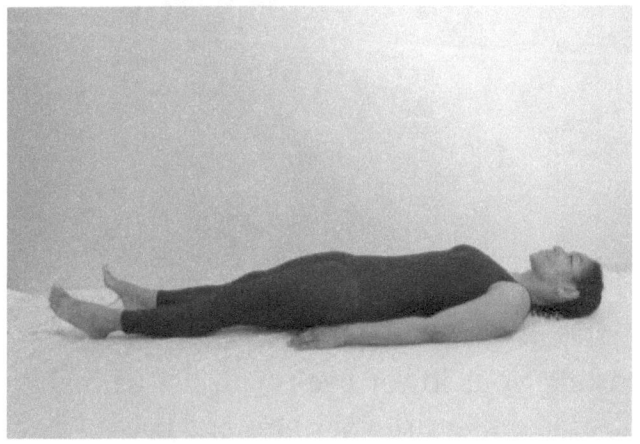

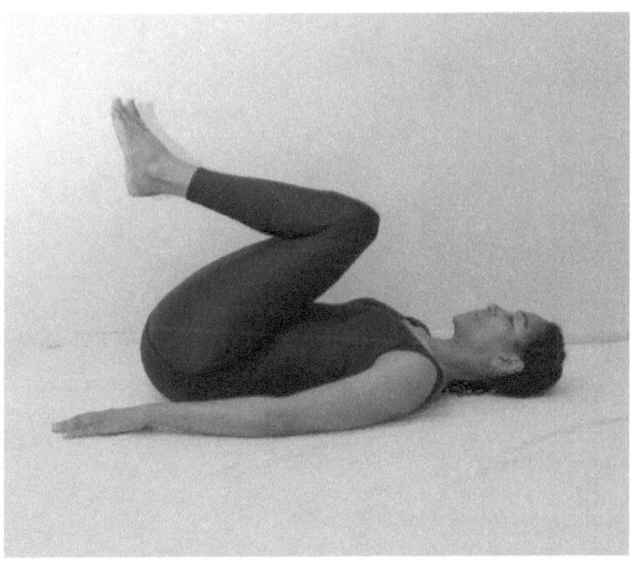

Bring your knees up over your chest.

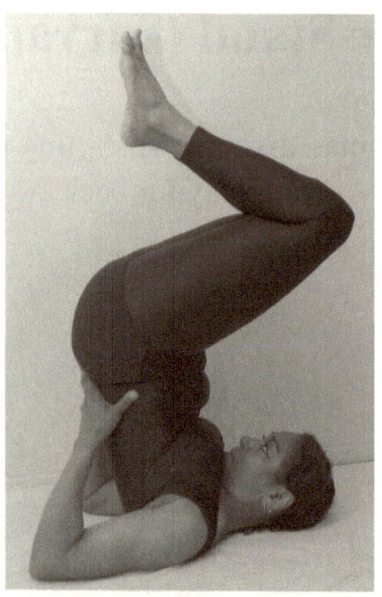

Supporting your lower back with the palms of your hands, gradually raise your hips and back.

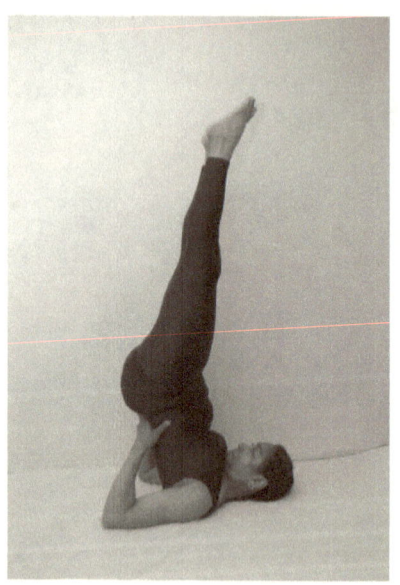

Lift your legs as high and as straight as you can. Rest your weight on your shoulders, keeping your elbows as close together as possible. Keep your legs straight, supporting your back with the palms of your hands. Look up at your feet. This posture can be held for one minute if you are a beginner. If you are comfortable, it can be held for up to three minutes or longer.

Supporting your lower back, slowly lower your upper body to your mat. Your legs may be bent or straight.

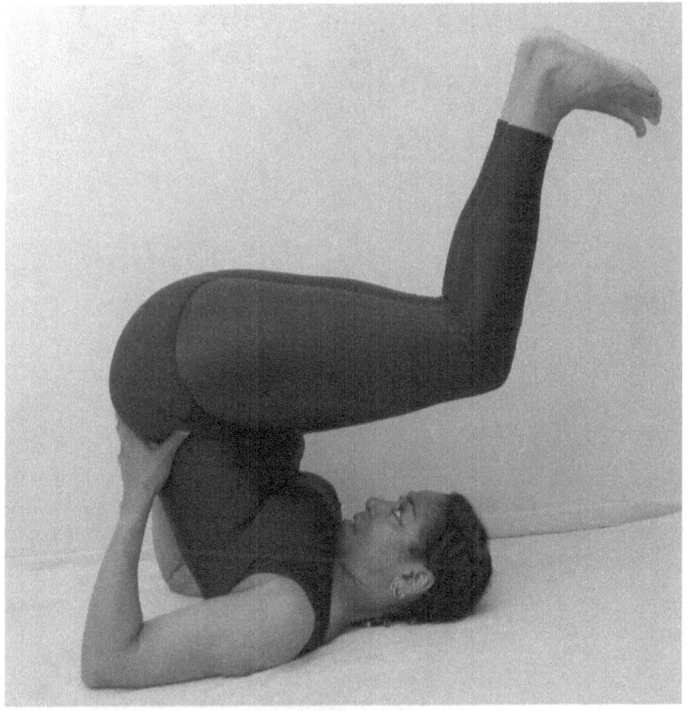

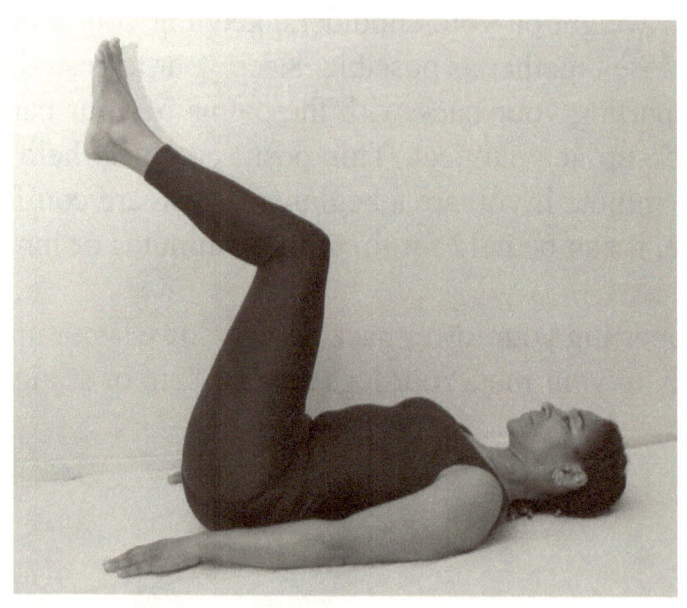

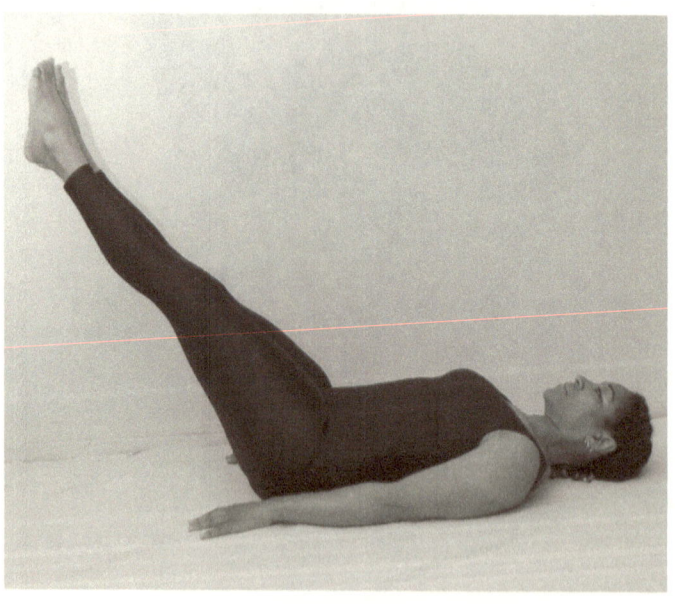

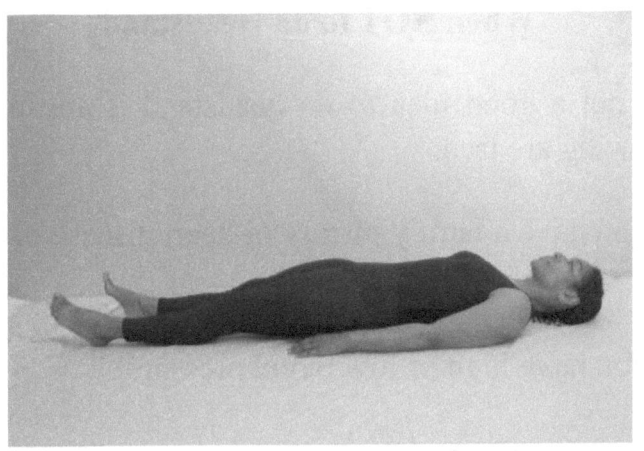

Benefits of Shoulder Stand

The shoulder stand rests the heart by using gravity to stimulate the circulation of blood to the brain.
Practicing the shoulder stand can lower the blood
pressure and bring it to normal.[7] The shoulder stand
calms the mind and relieves mild depression.

---

7   Krishna Raman, "Bio-Mechanics of Yoga," <www.
medicineau.net.au/columns/yoga/biomech.htm> .

When NOT to do Headstand

It is not a good idea to do headstand if any of the following are true:

- You have a family history of heart disease or stroke

- You have high or low blood pressure

- You are menstruating

- You have had a recent neck injury or have arthritis in your neck

- You are under thirteen years of age

- You have eye problems, such as cataracts or a detached retina

Headstand (Sirshasana)

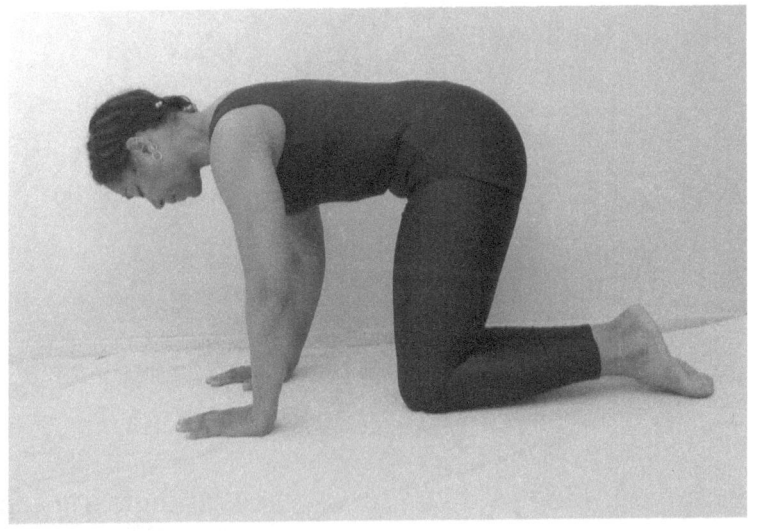

Come to your hands and knees on your mat
with your legs together.

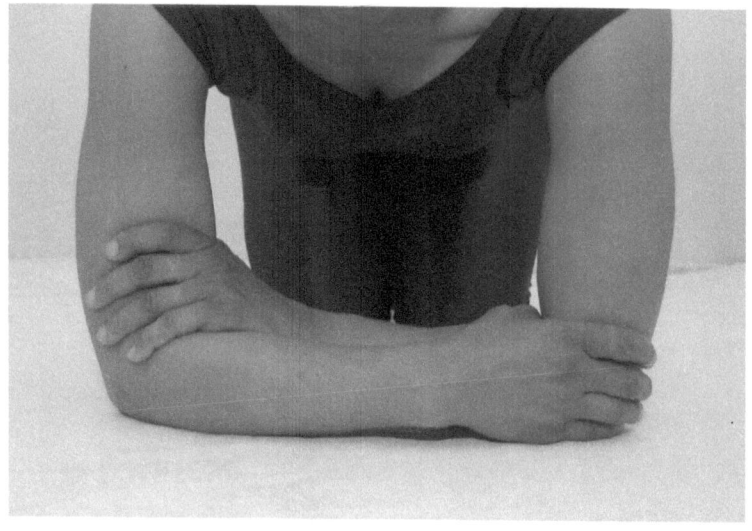

Bring your elbows down to your mat and grasp each elbow with the opposite hand to set the distance of your arms.

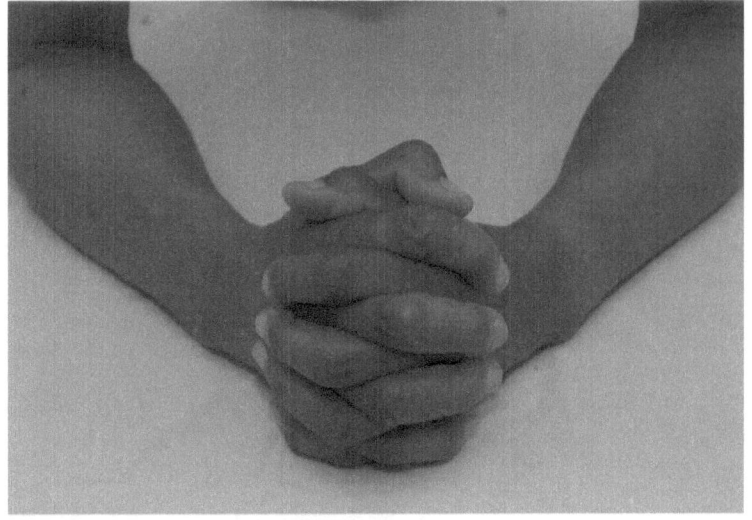

Extend your forearms and interlace your fingers to form a triangular base for your headstand.

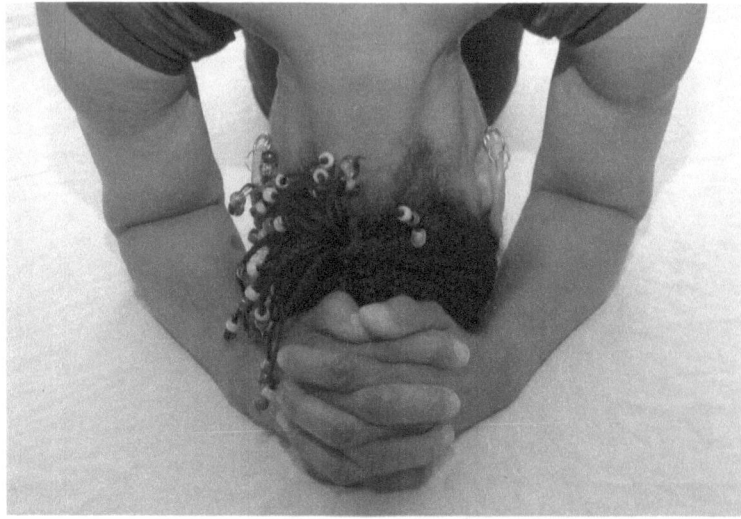

Place the top of your head down on your mat, so that the interlaced fingers are supporting the back of your head. Press your elbows firmly into your mat at all times throughout this pose.

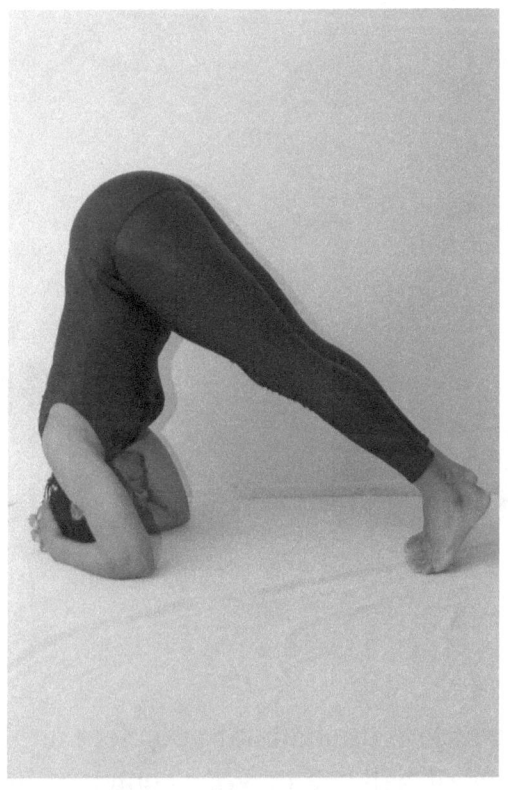

Straighten your legs into a jackknife position.

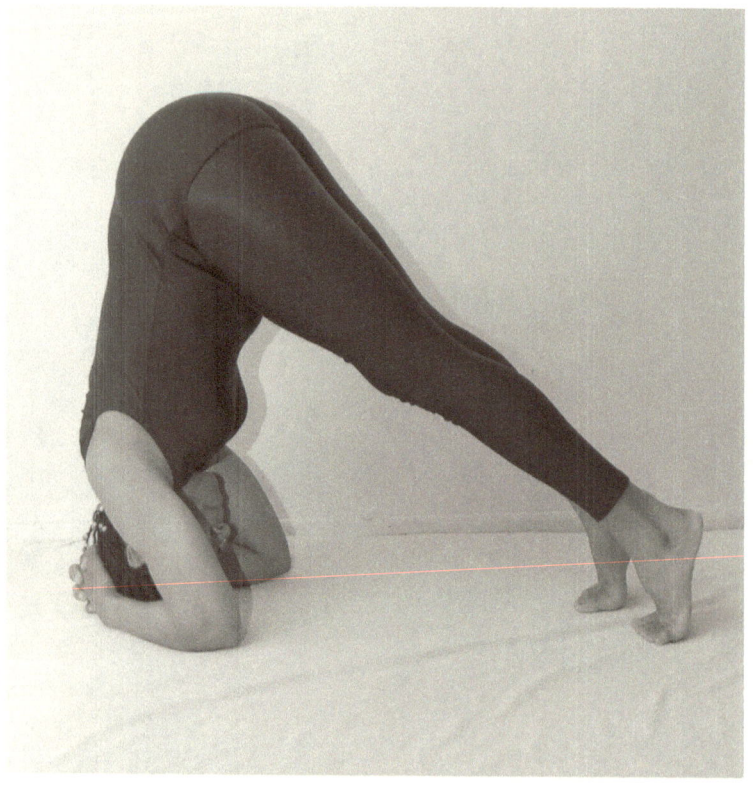

Walk forward on the balls of your feet until you find your center of balance or your center of gravity. Do not proceed any further until you have found this center. If you do not proceed beyond this point, you have already achieved a full inversion of the brain and the heart.

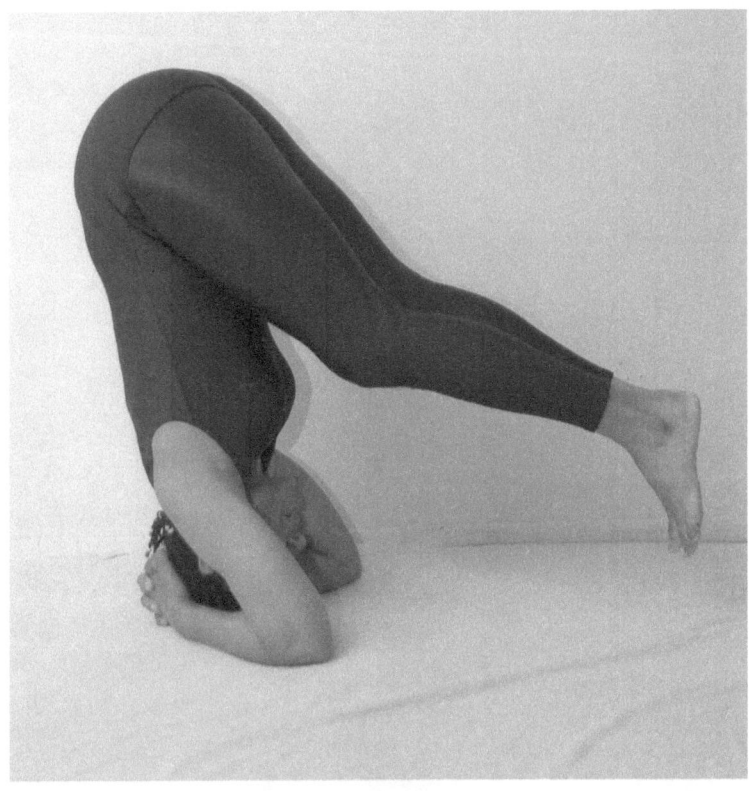

Maintaining this center, slowly lift your toes off your mat, bending your knees slightly.

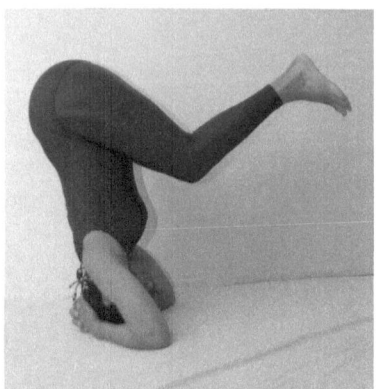

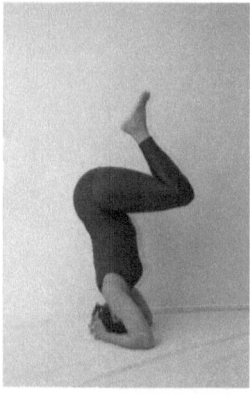

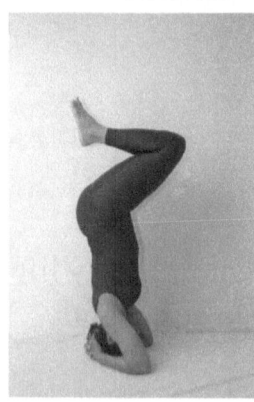

Keeping your knees as close to your body as possible, gradually raise your legs upward until they are straight. Press your elbows firmly into your mat.

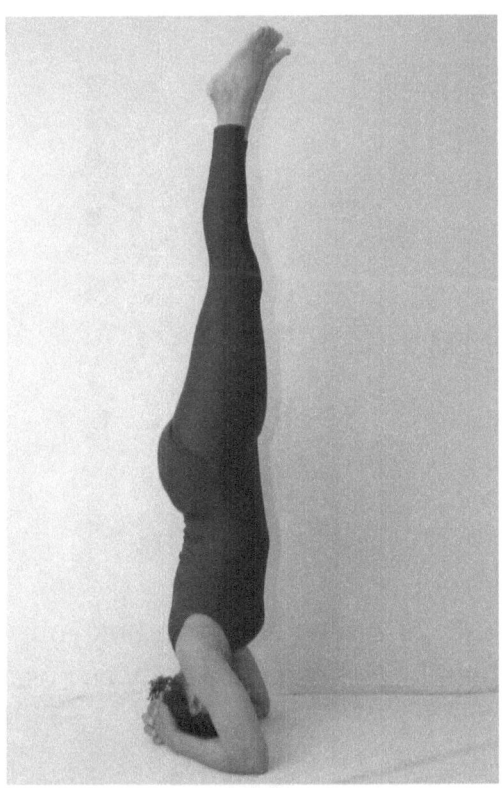

Hold this pose for one minute, if you are a beginner. The ideal time to hold this pose is three minutes.[8]

---

8   Jess Stearn, *Yoga, Youth & Reincarnation*, 288.

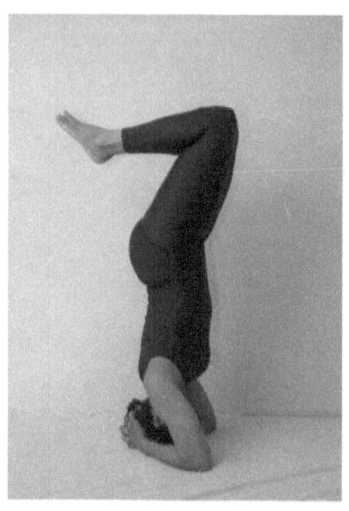

Lower your legs gradually by bending your knees and keeping them as close to your body as possible.

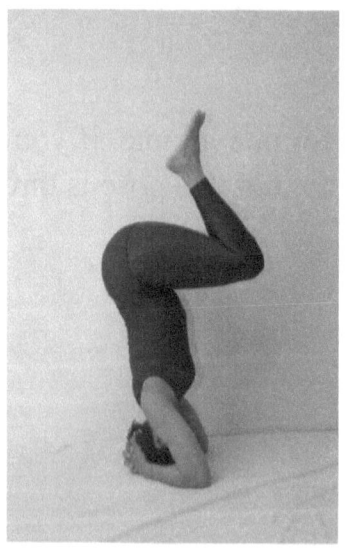

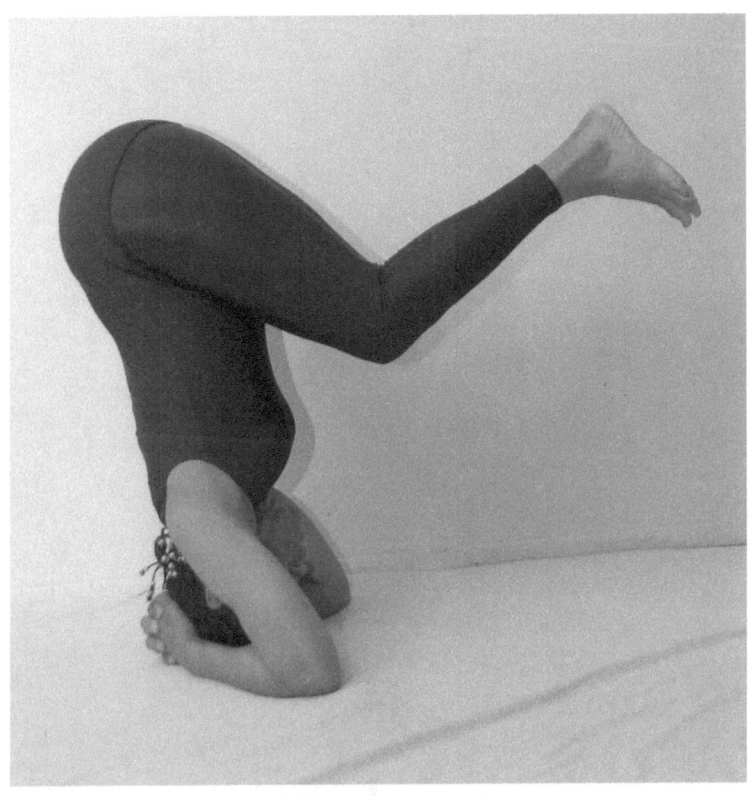

Lower your legs back into the jackknife position.

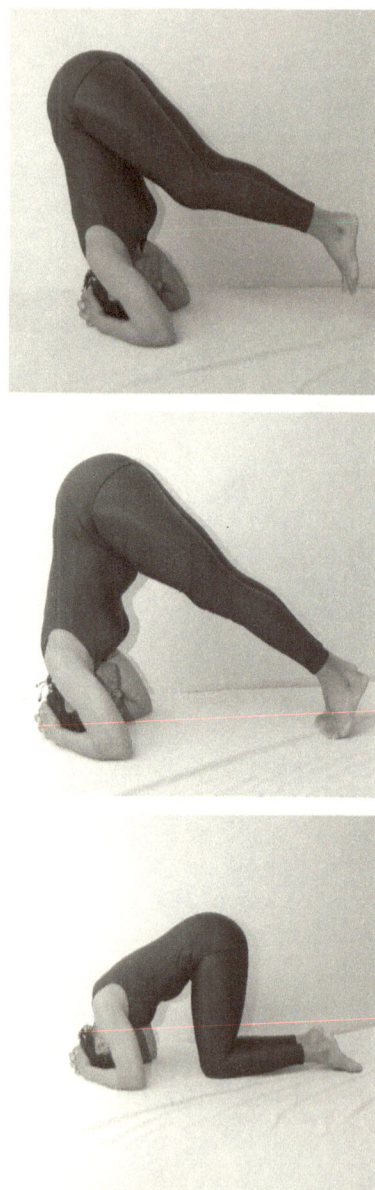

From the jackknife position, come down to your knees, leaving your elbows down and your fingers interlaced and supporting the back of your head.

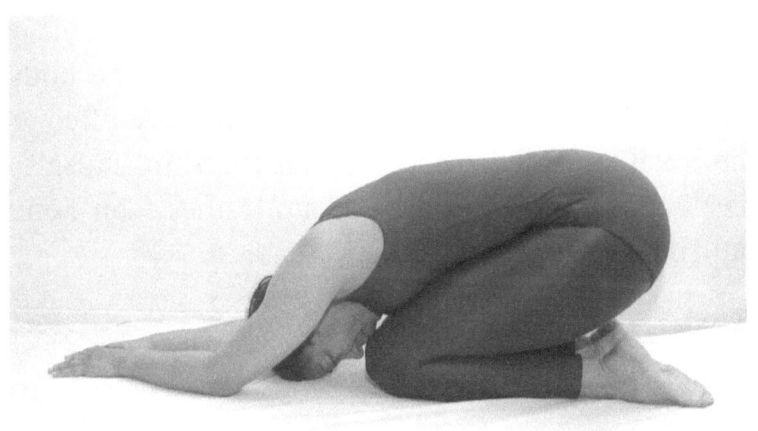

Sit back on your heels, allowing your chest to rest on your thighs. Place your forehead on your mat, stretching your arms out in front of you. Remain in this rest position for two minutes before standing upright. This position of rest, the child pose (Balasana), allows the body to assimilate the benefits of this inversion and allows the circulation of the blood to normalize.[9]

Benefits of Headstand

The headstand improves the circulation of blood to the brain. It also lowers the blood pressure. It improves concentration, memory, and mental alertness and calms the mind. The headstand relieves depression and promotes self-confidence.[10] It improves

---

9   Srivatsa Ramaswami, *Yoga for the Three Stages of Life*, 142 and 144.
10   Jess Stearn, *Yoga, Youth & Reincarnation*, 289.

the complexion and reduces wrinkles.[11] The pull of gravity continues during the inversion of the body, but the effects are reversed. The cumulative effect of the inversion of the body is that the skin, muscles, tissues, and organs are lifted up, rather than being pulled down.

---

11   Toby Hempel, *The New Yoga*, 40-41.

Inversion Therapy Devices

There are many inversion therapy devices available on the market. The most common inversion therapy device is the inversion table. The inversion table can be adjusted to various angles, allowing partial to full inversion of the body. Some of the benefits of this inversion therapy device are: heightened mental alertness due to an increased blood flow to the brain, relief from depression, and a youthful complexion.[12]

When NOT to Use Inversion Therapy

The following is a generalized[13] list of contraindications for the use of inversion therapy:

You have had a recent head injury
- You have fainting spells
- You have had an acute spinal injury

12   Wayne Franson, "Benefits of Inversion Therapy," < www.backandbodysolutions.com/inversion.html>.
13   Ibid.

- You are disoriented when upside down
- You have a detached retina
- You have cerebral sclerosis
- You have had a recent stroke

Consult your doctor before using an inversion therapy device if you have any of the following conditions:

- Glaucoma
- High blood pressure
- Recent back injury
- Chronic sinusitis
- You are being treated for heart and circulatory disorders

Conclusion

There is a tendency to react to things that we see. We have seen the effect of the invisible force of gravity on our bodies with the passage of time. It is urgent that we take a proactive rather than a reactive approach to the forces of gravity and time, by partly or completely inverting the brain and the heart. When the brain is positioned below the heart for a few minutes daily, the negative forces of gravity and time can be greatly reduced. Think of it (the inversion of the brain and heart) as your brain receiving its daily vitamins in fresh blood from the heart. Give your brain its daily dose! Your brain has neurotransmitters, like a complex machine. The blood supply that the brain receives from the heart during the inversion of the brain and heart can be considered as fuel to keep the neurotransmitters up and running. When the brain and heart are inverted, they can work together more efficiently. The mild, (or partial), inversion of the brain and heart can be achieved by anyone, and *everyone* is entitled to its benefits. The entire body is invigorated, and the aging process is delayed. The inversion of the brain and heart is eternally essential. It is never too late. The time to act is now!

References

Farhi, Donna. *Yoga Mind, Body & Spirit: A Return to Wholeness*. New York, New York: Henry Holt and Company, 2000.

Franson, Wayne. "Benefits of Inversion Therapy," *Inversion Therapy*. <www.backandbodysolutions.com/inversion.html> (accessed 01 April, 2009).

Hempel, Toby. *The New Yoga*. Boca Raton, Florida: Globe Communications Corp., 1985.

Powell, Lenore. Ed. D., with Katie Courtice. *Alzheimer's Disease: A Guide for Families and Caregivers, Third Edition*. Cambridge, Massachusetts: Perseus Publishing, 2002.

Raman, Krishna. "Bio-Mechanics of Yoga," *Biodynamics of Yoga*. <www.medicineau.net.au/

columns/yoga/biomech.htm> (accessed 27 January 2009).

Ramaswami, Srivatsa. *Yoga for the Three Stages of Life*. Rochester, Vermont: Inner Traditions, 2000.

Sabbagh, Marwan Noel. *The Alzheimer's Answer*. Hoboken, New Jersey: John Wiley & Sons, Inc., 2008.

Stearn, Jess. *Yoga, Youth & Reincarnation*. New York, New York: Doubleday & Company, Inc., 1965.

About the Author

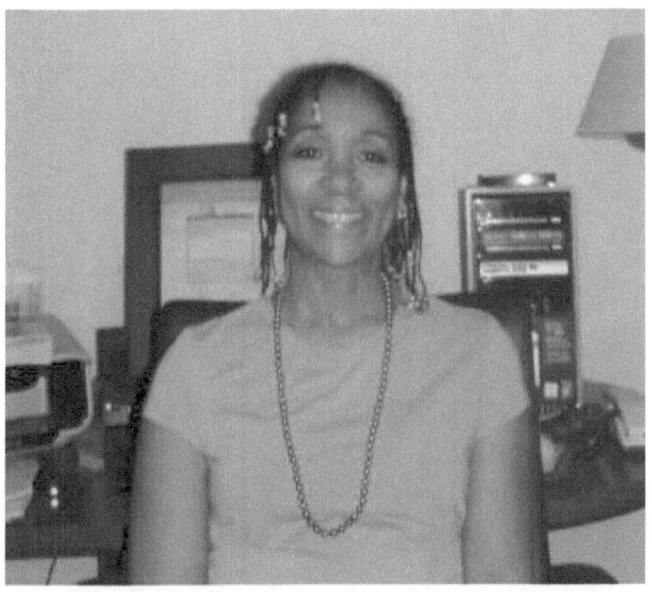

Carol Curtis was born in Albion, Michigan, the United States, and educated in Toronto, Ontario, Canada. She has been an elementary and secondary school teacher for the Toronto District School Board for over thirty years. She has been practicing yoga for more than twenty-five years. Swimming is also her passion.